Camila Dias de Farias
Maria Amélia A. S. Costa
José Jackson do N. Costa

Anti-inflammatory and healing effects of Vitamin E

Camila Dias de Farias
Maria Amélia A. S. Costa
José Jackson do N. Costa

Anti-inflammatory and healing effects of Vitamin E

Development of an educational booklet

ScienciaScripts

Imprint

Cover image: www.ingimage.com

This book is a translation from the original published under ISBN 978-620-2-40313-9.

Publisher:
Sciencia Scripts
is a trademark of
Dodo Books Indian Ocean Ltd. and OmniScriptum S.R.L publishing group

120 High Road, East Finchley, London, N2 9ED, United Kingdom
Str. Armeneasca 28/1, office 1, Chisinau MD-2012, Republic of Moldova, Europe
Printed at: see last page
ISBN: 978-620-8-30443-0

PRESENTATION

Dear readers,

This book is part of the results achieved by the author Camila Dias de Farias, in the development of her Course Conclusion Work, in the Bachelor's Degree course in Nutrition at the Instituto Superior de Teologia Aplicada - INTA.

The work was conceived taking into account the importance of vitamin E in the protection and regeneration of epithelial tissue, as well as its effects in blocking cellular oxidation and eliminating free radicals which become very aggressive to cells when in excess in the body. Its role in the treatment of pathologies such as cancer, atherosclerosis, hypertension and skin wounds can be highlighted. Vitamin E is a fat-soluble antioxidant that has a potentially anti-inflammatory and healing effect on skin wounds.

There is also the need to create educational materials that can bring all this information to the target public and the need to use them in instructional interventions, communicating content produced for health education that is available in the PSF. It's worth noting the growing existence of educational materials in the PSF. However, most of the time these materials come with tiresome texts and a lot of technical terms that end up losing the interest of the target audience.

The creation of materials on the anti-inflammatory and healing function of vitamin E is therefore favorable, based on the need for new studies and results that can further improve knowledge about the characteristics of vitamin E.

SUMMARY

The aim of this study was to produce an explanatory booklet emphasizing the anti-inflammatory and healing effects of vitamin E. To achieve these objectives, a bibliographic and qualitative study was carried out, targeting patients with diabetes, the elderly, bedridden individuals and health professionals from the Family Health Program. The process of creating the booklet was based on the principles of educational-dialogical practice, helping users of public health services to change their lifestyle. Readers will have the opportunity to broaden their understanding of the problem and reflect on the importance of vitamin E. The selection and use of illustrations in the booklet facilitates understanding and comprehension by the target audience. This work demonstrated some of the beneficial effects of vitamin E in patients with various types of inflammatory processes. This highlighted the importance of eating a diet rich in vitamin E, given its fundamental role in antioxidant, anti-inflammatory and healing processes. As for the booklet, it was designed using simple language, in a didactic way, with the aim of avoiding too many pages, always aiming for the best understanding on the part of the users, as well as the acquisition of knowledge about the subjects covered. In conclusion, the educational experience using the booklet can be an important means of informing, building knowledge and promoting reflection on the benefits of vitamin E.

Keywords: Anti-inflammatory. Antioxidant. Healing. Vitamin E.

SUMMARY

1. INTRODUCTION

Organisms have adaptive mechanisms to respond to aggressive stimuli in order to maintain homeostatic balance, including a series of biochemical, physiological and immunological alterations collectively known as inflammation (VOLTARELLI, 1994; LOPES, 2011). Inflammation is a defense response that occurs after cell damage caused by microorganisms, characterized by the production of inflammatory mediators and the movement of liquid and leukocytes from the blood to the tissues. Through these mechanisms, the body locates and eliminates altered cells, foreign particles or micro-organisms through metabolic processes (LIMA *et al.,* 2007).

Inflammation can be divided into an acute phase and a chronic phase. In an attempt to defend the body against injury, in the acute phase, a regulatory reaction arises which is the Systemic Inflammatory Response Syndrome (SIRS). SIRS is characterized by catabolism, weight loss and even malnutrition, compromising immune functions and healing. There is also an increase in the production of inflammatory mediators, an increase in endocrine secretions, the production of reactive oxygen species (ROS) and an imbalance in the level of antioxidants (GUYTON; HALL, 2006). Among the substances that reduce inflammation are antioxidants, which are a heterogeneous set of elements made up of vitamins, minerals, natural pigments and other plant compounds, as well as enzymes, which block the damaging effect of free radicals that contribute to various inflammatory reactions and hinder the healing process (MESSIAS, 2009). In this context, vitamins, especially vitamin E, stand out as antioxidants.

Vitamins are organic substances present in many foods in small quantities, but which are indispensable for the functioning of the body in the form of cofactors. Vitamins can be classified into into fat-soluble and water-soluble (PAIXAO; STAMFORD, 2004). The role of vitamin E, also known as alpha-tocopherol (a-tocopherol), which is fat-soluble and has solubility characteristics similar to those of lipids, stands out in the inflammatory process. The main metabolic function of vitamin E is its antioxidant action, capable of interrupting the chain of reactions characteristic of lipid peroxidation. Its absorption occurs in the lumen of the small intestine in a process dependent on bile and pancreatic secretions (PHILIPPI, 2012). The main sources of vitamin E in the human diet are oils (soybean, corn, linseed, cottonseed, canola, palm, sesame, wheat germ, peanut, sunflower, olive); margarines (corn, soybean, sunflower); seeds (sesame, sunflower); nuts (almond, peanut, Brazil nut); cereal grains (corn, rice) (ARAUJO *et al.,* 2003).

The lack of knowledge on the part of patients is one of the aspects to be considered, so health professionals are responsible for encouraging the process of acquiring knowledge and possible changes in the control of various diseases, such as the inflammatory process (MONETTA, 1990). In this way, health education practices should be included in all the support developed within the SUS. Providing an interaction between the objectives of the SUS and its beneficiaries, with perspectives of social participation, understanding that true educational practices only take place between social subjects (BRASIL, 2007).

Health education and its interfaces in health promotion have dimensions that include political, social and cultural issues, as well as involving the practical and theoretical aspects of individuals and their communities. It also encompasses the concepts of education and health, as well as the health-disease process. It is therefore considered an important tool for health promotion (SALCI *etal.,* 2013).

In view of the above, it is understood that education for participation in health emphasizes man as the main subject and the following problem arises: what is the need for an educational booklet that emphasizes the nutritional importance of vitamin E?

2. CHAPTER 1 - LITERATURE REVIEW

2.1 Inflammation and the immune system

Inflammation, also known as the inflammatory process, is the body's natural response to infection or injury, with the aim of expelling and destroying foreign cells that are considered to be aggressive agents. The causes of inflammation can be of biological origin involving agents such as bacteria, viruses or parasites, or of chemical origin involving factors such as poison, heat, exposure to radiation or trauma (GOLDMAN; AUSIELLO, 2009).

According to Guyton and Hall (2006), when an organ is injured or infected, inflammatory mediators, such as histamine, are released, giving rise to the inflammatory response. The mediators increase blood supply to the site of injury, stimulate the production of other inflammatory substances that increase the permeability of blood vessels and also chemotaxis (a chemical process by which blood cells such as neutrophils and macrophages are attracted to the site of injury). These cells will destroy the agents causing the inflammation and produce chemical substances that activate platelets to control possible bleeding. All these supports are part of the immune system (GUYTON; HALL, 2006). The immune system and its collective and coordinated response to the introduction of foreign cells is called the immune response.

Inflammation is part of natural immunity, also called innate or native immunity. The main components of the natural immune system are physical and chemical barriers, such as epithelium and antibacterial substances, phagocytic cells such as neutrophils and macrophages and *natural killer* cells, blood proteins, including fractions of the complement system, mediators, etc.

of inflammation and proteins called cytokines. In contrast to natural immunity, there is adaptive or acquired immunity which occurs through stimulation and exposure to infectious agents (ROITT; DELVES, 2004).

The inflammatory process can be classified as acute or chronic, depending on the intensity and time it takes for the symptoms to appear and be fought off, and the type of cells and antibodies present in the area of the injury. The inflammatory process has three main stages, which are changes in vascular flow and caliber, increased vascular permeability or vascular extravasation and the emigration of leukocytes from the microcirculation and their accumulation in the lesion focus (LIMA *et al.,* 2007).

In acute inflammation there are first changes in vascular flow and caliber, where vasodilation occurs after an inconstant and transient vasoconstriction of the arterioles, lasting a few seconds. There is an increase in blood flow, which generates heat and erythema. This is followed by an increase in vascular permeability, resulting in the extravasation of a protein-rich liquid into the interstitium, known as exudate, which is the hallmark of acute inflammation (FERREIRA *etal.,* 2006). As inflammation sets in, some signs and symptoms may appear, such as heat, redness or flushing, swelling or edema and pain. These signs are typical of an inflammatory process, especially when it is acute inflammation. If not resolved in time, inflammation can lead to loss of function of the inflamed organ or tissue (GUYTON; HALL, 2006).

The physiological function of the immune system is defense against infectious micro-organisms, i.e. external invaders (antigens) (FILHO; BOGLIOLO, 2009). The broadest definition of immunity would be a reaction to foreign substances, including micro-organisms and macromolecules such as proteins and polysaccharides, and to small chemical substances that are recognized as foreign elements, regardless of the physiological and pathological consequences of such a reaction. The immune system plays an important role in the production of vaccines, in cell culture techniques including antibodies (SILVA; MOTA, 2003).

The pharmacological treatment of inflammation can be carried out through corticosteroids, such as prednisolone or prednisone, used mainly to treat chronic inflammation; or through the use of non-steroidal anti-inflammatory drugs, such as ibuprofen or acetylsalicylic acid, used mainly to treat acute inflammation. During the inflammatory process, inflammatory mediators are released, which are responsible for giving rise to the different phases of inflammation. Some mediators are histamine, cytokines and platelet activating factors (GOLDMAN; AUSIELLO, 2009).

Among the cells of the immune system that participate in the inflammatory process, macrophages and B lymphocytes stand out. Macrophages are important in regulating the immune response. They are present in connective tissues and in the blood, where they are called monocytes. In the immune system, macrophages have the function of detecting and phagocytizing antigens. The main function of B lymphocytes is to produce antibodies when they are mature and active (ROITT *et al.,* 2003). The immune system is made up of two groups of immune organs, which participate in the production and maturation of lymphocytes. The primary immune organs are: the bone marrow, which produces B lymphocytes and *natural killer* cells; and the secondary immune organs are the lymph nodes, which are present in the lymphatic vessels, where the lymph is filtered, allowing invading particles to be phagocytosed by the lymphocytes present (FILHO; BOGLIOLO, 2009).

2.2 Cellular oxidation and inflammation

Oxidative stress is due to excess production of oxidants (free radicals) or depletion of antioxidant defenses. According to Ferreira and Matsubara (1997), free radicals are: an atom or molecule that has a They have an odd number of electrons in the last electron layer, are unstable and highly reactive, so they are always trying to capture or give up electrons from the cells around them, whose unpaired electrons are centered on the oxygen or nitrogen atoms, forming reactive oxygen species (ROS) or reactive nitrogen species (RNS), respectively (FERREIRA; MATSUBARA, 1997). In the body, RLs are involved in energy production, phagocytosis, cell growth regulation, intercellular signaling and the synthesis of important biological substances (BARREIROS *et al.,* 2006).

The excess of free radicals in the body is combated by antioxidants produced by the body or absorbed from the diet (BARREIROS *et al.*, 2006). Their production can be beneficial in cases of infection, when RLs are produced by phagocytic cells to kill invading microorganisms, or harmful when inflammation becomes systemic, as in the case of sepsis, where loss of control of RL production can cause distant damage (MONTERA, 2007). According to Barbosa *et al.* (2014), antioxidants such as ascorbate (AsA), glutathione (GSH), p-carotene and a-tocopherol can prevent the formation of free radicals, as well as sequester them or promote their degradation, preventing damage to plant cells.

In the process of reducing molecular oxygen, ROS are formed and these free radicals need to be permanently inactivated. Free radicals can affect many biological molecules, including lipids, proteins, carbohydrates and vitamins present in food. ROS are also implicated in various human diseases. There is evidence that a diet rich in antioxidants reduces the risk of the main human diseases, such as cardiovascular diseases, neurodegenerative diseases, cancer and the ageing process (BIANCHI and ANTUNES, 1999; PEREIRA *et al.,* 2009).

In the case of exacerbated production of RLs, the body has an efficient antioxidant system that can control and restore balance. Oxidative stress results from an imbalance between the pro- and antioxidant systems, with oxidants predominating. The cell is a veritable powerhouse of pro- and antioxidants (VASCONCELOS *etal.,* 2007).

RLs can be generated in clinical situations where microenvironments of hypoxia are followed by microenvironments of reoxygenation (JUNIOR *et al.,* 2005), causing alterations in biomolecules such as proteins, carbohydrates, lipids and deoxyribonucleic acid. According to Ramalho and Jorge (2006), lipids, for example, can be oxidized by different routes such as hydrolytic reactions catalyzed by lipase enzymes or by the action of heat and humidity, with the formation of free fatty acids. Enzymatic oxidation occurs through the action of lipoxygenase enzymes which act on polyunsaturated fatty acids, catalyzing the addition of oxygen to the polyunsaturated hydrocarbon chain.

Treatment with antioxidants seems promising in mitigating the effects of uncontrolled production of LRs in critically ill patients; however, there is a lack of evidence defining the best form of supplementation and the appropriate stage of the disease for this. The adverse effects of their clinical use must also be taken into account, as all antioxidants can have a pro-oxidant effect and increase tissue damage. Therefore, considering the risks of deficiency, but also of excess, one should try not to exceed the recommended amounts and combinations of micronutrients (LEITE; SARNI, 2003).

Due to more recent knowledge of the role of immunological and inflammatory mechanisms, as well as oxidative stress in the pathophysiology of inflammatory disease, much of this effort has been focused on therapies, mainly drugs, that can control these mechanisms (BARREIROS *et al.,* 2006).

ROS, which can originate either exogenously or endogenously, are also produced during pathological processes, such as what occurs in a cellular inflammatory response. ROS is a broad term that covers not only oxygen radicals, but also other radicals (BERRA *et al.,* 2006). Interest in the mechanisms of oxygen free radical (OFR) generation and adaptation to exercise has increased significantly since their relationship with oxygen consumption was demonstrated. RLOs are formed by the incomplete reduction of oxygen, generating species that are highly reactive towards other biomolecules, mainly lipids and cell membrane proteins, and even DNA (SCHNEIDER and OLIVEIRA, 2004). However, it is now known that adequate nutritional support, with modulation of micronutrients with antioxidant activity or which act as cofactors for antioxidant elements, is capable of reducing oxidative stress and the inflammatory process.

According to Pereira *et al.* (2009) antioxidants in the diet can produce an effective protective action against the oxidative processes that occur in the body. Among natural antioxidants, fruits and vegetables are the foods that contribute most to the dietary supply of these compounds. Thus, the action of antioxidants such as vitamin C, vitamin E, phenolic compounds and carotenoids has stimulated intense research.

According to Montera (2007) immunological, inflammatory and oxidative stress mechanisms play a significant role in the development and progression of chronic inflammation. According to Junior *et al.* (2001) there is an incidence of diseases related to carcinogenic processes in the body, involving the formation of reactive oxygen species such as hydrogen peroxide and the hydroxyl radical, there is a relationship between glutathione levels, acting directly or indirectly in many important biological processes, including protein synthesis, metabolism and cell protection.

While antioxidants include enzymes that minimize the availability of pro-oxidants (BERRA *et al.,* 2006).

The damage caused by oxidative stress has cumulative effects and is related to a number of diseases, such as cancer, atherosclerosis and diabetes (SCHNEIDER; OLIVEIRA, 2004). Junior *et al.* (2005), indicate that there is also an influence of RLOs on the main lung diseases caused by cigarette use, such as chronic obstructive pulmonary disease (COPD), asthma, obstructive sleep apnea and acute respiratory distress syndrome (SCHNEIDER; OLIVEIRA, 2004).

Problems in the synthesis and metabolism of glutathione are

associated with some diseases, in which the levels of glutathione and the enzymes that act in its metabolism can be very significant in the diagnosis of some types of cancer, as well as in other diseases related to oxidative stress, such as rheumatoid arthritis and myocardial oxidative stress (JUNIOR *et al.*, 2001).

2.3 Vitamin E

Vitamins are biologically active organic nutrients needed by the body to maintain vital processes. Deficiencies of vitamins lead to so-called deficiency diseases. Vitamins can be classified as water-soluble vitamins, which are soluble in water; and fat-soluble vitamins, which are soluble in fats and are absorbed in the human intestine with the help of bile salts secreted by the liver (PENTEADO, 2003).

The body can store a greater quantity of fat-soluble vitamins than water-soluble ones. Vitamin E is stored in fatty tissues and, to a lesser extent, in the reproductive organs. The main sources of vitamin E in the human diet are oils (soybean, corn, linseed, cottonseed, canola, palm, sesame, wheat germ, peanut, sunflower, olive); margarines (corn, soybean, sunflower); seeds (sesame, sunflower); nuts (almond, pecan, peanut, Brazil nut); cereal grains (corn, rice) (ARAUJO *et al.,* 2003). It acts in the body as an inhibitor of oxidation processes in organic tissues. It protects unsaturated fats from oxidation by peroxides or other free radicals (COSTA; ROSA, 2010).

Tocopherols and tocotrienois comprise at least 8 compounds with vitamin E activity. Only the (alpha)-tocopherol form (Figure 1) is maintained in human plasma. However, the activity of a-tocopherol *in vivo* is greater than that of the other compounds, being around 10 times greater than its immediate precursor, y-tocopherol. In addition, the absorption of tocopherols by the body is selective, and a-tocopherol predominates over the others (p, Y, and б-tocopherol), which are not absorbed or are absorbed only in small proportions (SOUSA *et al.,* 2007).

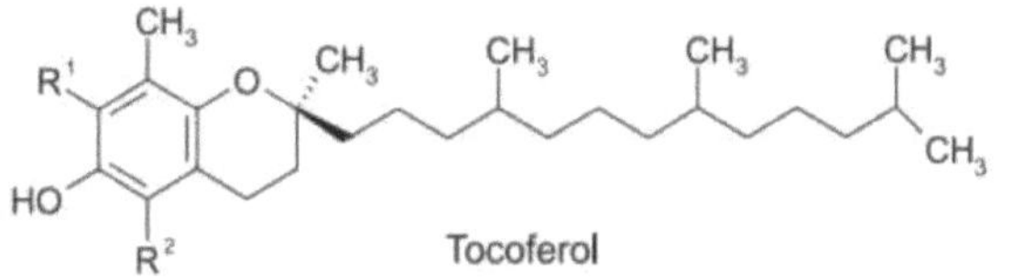

Tocoferol

Tocoferol	R^1	R^2
α-	CH_3	CH_3
β-	H	CH_3
γ-	CH_3	H
δ-	H	H

Figure 1: Chemical structure of tocopherol. Source: Adapted from Cerqueira;
Medeiros; Augusto, 2007.

During studies by Guinazi *et al.* (2009) with vegetable oils and raw and cooked egg yolks from commercial restaurants, it was shown that the composition of tocopherol and tocotrienol in foods varied considerably. Tocopherols were detected in greater quantity and frequency. A-tocopherol predominated in egg yolk and olive oil, while y-tocopherol was found in high quantities in soybean and canola oils. In addition, the cooking process of egg yolks did not cause major losses for most vitamin E isomers. According to Sousa *et al.* (2007), the nutritional value of tocopherols, in terms of vitamin E activity, is determined by the concentration of a-tocopherol. In this context, the importance of vitamin E is related to its antioxidant function which maintains the integrity of tissues, as well as playing important roles in biological processes (SOUSA *et al.,* 2007).

The Dietary Reference Intake (DRI) for vitamin E, according to US legislation (INSTITUTE OF MEDICINE, 2000) for men and women over 14 years of age and for pregnant women of any age is 15mg/day; for breastfeeding women it is 19mg/day. The DRIs for infants aged 0-6 months are 4mg/day; for children aged 1-3 years: 6mg/day; 4-8 years: 7mg/day; 9-13 years: 11mg/day and for those over 14 years 15mg/day (COZZOLINO, 2009).

Chestnuts contain phenolic acids and flavonoids, as well as being rich in tocopherols, phytosterols and squalene. They are a source of carbohydrates, essential fatty acids and minerals. Walnuts are high in n-3 fatty acids and low in saturated fatty acids, with high levels of vitamin E, polyphenols, flavonoids, arginine and fiber. The possible beneficial effects of these compounds are due to their antioxidant and antiproliferative activity, which are linked to a reduced risk of developing atherosclerosis and cancer (COSTA; JORGE, 2011).

TABLE 1. Main sources of vitamin E in the human diet.

Bread, cereals and other grains	Breakfast cereals Fortified cereals Wheat germ
Fruits	Baked map Apricot Raw nectarine Peach
Hortaligas	Chard Kale Mustard Courgette Turnip
Meat, poultry and substitutes	Liver, chicken or turkey
Fish	Canned seafood Boiled or baked corvina Pickled mackerel Baked or grilled salmon Baked or boiled scallop Boiled or baked shrimp

Nuts and seeds	Almond Walnuts Hazel Peanuts Peanut butter

Source: Penteado (2003)

Philippi (2008) points out that bioactive substances or compounds have a functional role that can provide health benefits, such as isoprenoids, phenolic compounds, fatty acids and essential amino acids, fibers, among others. Tocopherols are present in vegetables, especially in oil seeds, leaves, vegetable oils, fruit, nuts and cereals (PHILIPPI, 2008).

Fat-soluble vitamins, due to their complex metabolism, functional diversity and absorption mechanism related to lipoproteins, present some specific problems when it comes to assessing their bioavailability in foods or diets, requiring careful planning and analysis of results when carrying out tests (MOURAO *et al.,* 2005).

Once absorbed, vitamin E is incorporated into chylomicrons and thus reaches the liver. In the liver, a specific protein selectively chooses a-tocopherol from among the other tocopherols for incorporation into very low density lipoproteins (VLDLs). Thus, although the absorption process of all the tocopherol homologues in our diet is similar, the a-tocopherol form predominates in the blood and tissues (COSTA; ROSA, 2010).

Although the mechanisms involved in the absorption of alpha-tocopherol by the mammary gland are not completely clear, there is a consensus that a large part of the alpha-tocopherol reaches the milk via the traditional low-density lipoprotein (LDL) receptor pathway. Another part of vitamin E may be transported via cell surface receptors (SR-B1) that bind high- and low-density lipoproteins (HDL and LDL, respectively), without internalizing the lipoprotein (DIMENSTEIN *et al.,* 2011).

2.3.1 Anti-inflammatory effect of vitamin E

Vitamin E's ability to modulate signal transduction and gene expression has been observed in several studies. However, the detailed molecular mechanisms involved are often unclear. The eight natural analogues of vitamin E and their synthetic derivatives affect signal transduction with different potency, possibly reflecting their different ability to interact with specific proteins (ZINGG, 2007).

There is evidence that vitamin E plays an important role in modulating prostaglandin synthesis and, consequently, platelet aggregation. It has been observed that lipid peroxidation occurs during the platelet aggregation process (COSTA; ROSA, 2010).

The study by Zingg (2007) reports that the main effects of vitamin E on the enzymes involved in signal transduction are yet to be summarized and the possible mechanisms leading to this modulation need to be better evaluated. Elucidating the molecular and cellular events affected by vitamin E could reveal new strategies and molecular targets for the development of compounds that act in the same way.

In this context, a-tocopherol modulates two main signal transduction pathways centered on protein kinase C and phosphatidylinositol-3-kinase. Alterations in the activity of these main kinases are associated with changes in cell proliferation, platelet aggregation and NADPH-oxidase activation. Several genes are also regulated by tocopherols, partly due to the effects of tocopherol on these two kinases, but also independently (AZZI *etal.,* 2006).

Zingg (2007) indicates that vitamin E modulates the activity of several enzymes involved in signal transduction, such as protein kinase C, protein kinase B, protein tyrosine kinases, 5-, 12- and 15-lipoxygenases, cyclooxygenase-2, phospholipase A2, protein phosphatase 2A, protein tyrosine phosphatase, and diacylglycerol kinase. The activation of some of

these enzymes after stimulation of cell surface receptors with growth factors or cytokines can be normalized by vitamin E (ZINGG, 2007). However, it is known that adequate nutritional support, with the modulation of micronutrients with antioxidant activity or that act as cofactors for antioxidant elements, is capable of reducing oxidative stress and the inflammatory process, mainly by modulating 20
gene transcription responsible for generating a response to extracellular stimuli or modifying the cell's internal environment (MONTERA, 2007).

In a study, Bertagnon *et al.* (2014) used alpha tocopherol and found a potential improvement in the defense system, where it was observed that alpha tocopherol reduced cellular oxidative stress, increasing phagocytosis and oxidative metabolism of neutrophils, and decreased lipoperoxidation of cell membranes by increasing the half-life of blood cells.

2.3.2 Antioxidant effect of vitamin E

In the human diet there are various sources of nutrients with an antioxidant role, capable of preventing or minimizing cardiovascular effects and diabetic complications. Alpha-tocopherol stands out due to its mechanisms of action and its food sources. However, proper nutrition is the best alternative for a quality life, since researchers claim that meeting daily antioxidant needs can prevent or treat chronic non-communicable diseases (ZIMMERMANN; KIRSTEN, 2008).

The antioxidant action of vitamin E can also be highlighted. Studies on oxidative stress in neonates by Nogueira *et al.* (2010) show that oxidative stress is present in neonates, especially premature infants, increasing the demand for antioxidant nutrients. There is a consensus that these should be administered in combination in order to prevent cell damage. Longitudinal studies with larger sample sizes are needed to assess the concentrations of these antioxidant micronutrients in order to draw up appropriate recommendations for term and preterm neonates (NOGUEIRA *et al.*, 2010).

The methods for evaluating total antioxidant activity (TAA) proposed in the literature are diverse, but some are more appropriate than others, depending on the nature of the compounds present in the composition of each fruit. It evaluates the antioxidant activity of fruit in order to monitor the methodological progress of the main antioxidant tests currently in use (SUCUPIRA *et al.*, 2012).

Nutritional therapy with antioxidants concomitant with the administration of antineoplastic drugs has several benefits for the treatment of cancer patients. The supply of antioxidant vitamins such as A, E and C associated with antiblastic drugs results in fewer side effects and allows the continuity of the treatment used not to be jeopardized, since the toxicity caused by antineoplastic drugs is a limiting factor of this therapy (SANTOS; CRUZ, 2001).

Chronic non-communicable diseases can be aggravated by oxidative stress, which is an imbalance between reactive oxygen species and the capacity of antioxidants to act. To reduce the damage caused by oxidative stress, dietary antioxidants act as suicide molecules, neutralizing the free radical (ZIMMERMANN; KIRSTEN, 2008).

The supply of antioxidant vitamins such as A, C and E has benefits for the prevention of cervical cancer, especially in the early stages of cervical carcinogenesis. Vitamin A, through its carotenoids, is able to inhibit the formation of free radicals and is also a powerful modulator of cell differentiation, which provides protection against the development of HPV. Vitamins C and E can prevent the formation of carcinogens and increase immunity (SAMPAIO; ALMEIDA, 2009).

Tocopherols, carotenoids and flavonoids, among others, have the function of preventing the attack of ROS and RNA or regenerating the damage caused to essential biological systems. The complex mechanism of the anti- and pro-oxidant activity of these substances is the subject of extensive contemporary scientific studies, since the success of these investigations is directly linked to related to improving human quality of life (BARREIROS *etal.,* 2005).

Sucupira *et al.* (2012) through studies involving antioxidant compounds naturally present in foods and the prevention or control of some non-communicable diseases have drawn the attention of the scientific community and the population in general. Among the foods that contain natural antioxidants, fruits and vegetables are the ones that contribute most to the dietary supply of these compounds, which are associated with beneficial effects on human health.

Nutritional therapy based on the use of antioxidants can broaden the concepts of current cancer therapy and enable better results in terms of cancer control. This article is a review of the literature, in which some aspects of the mechanism of drug action and the formation of free radicals arising from this will be described (SANTOS; CRUZ, 2001).

2.3.3 Vitamin E's healing effect

Wound healing is one of the fastest growing sectors in healthcare and pharmacists can make essential contributions (MORAIS *et al.,* 2013). The study of skin healing involves a huge range of events and special situations. It requires basic knowledge of anatomy, histology, biochemistry, immunology, pharmacology, among other sciences (MANDELBAUM *et al.,* 2003).

Among the substances used in wound treatment are sunflower oil, which stimulates cell proliferation, neoangiogenesis and acts as a pro-inflammatory mediator; propolis, which promotes an anti-inflammatory, bactericidal and healing action; papain, which aids in the degradation of granulation tissues and reduces debridement; d-panthenol, which stimulates skin protection, repair and renewal; and fibroblast growth factor, which indirectly promotes collagen synthesis and stimulates cell production and migration (MORAIS *et al.,* 2013). Due to the fact that there is a significant number of patients with chronic lesions or who have some kind of complication in the healing process, professionals involved in the treatments are required to be more knowledgeable and prepared to deal with this problem (MORAIS *et al.,* 2013).

In the study by Godoy and Prado (2005), wounds were mechanically or chemically debrided, followed by dressings in which essential fatty acids including enriched vitamin E were used as a topical substance, followed by occlusion with gauze. The substances allowed the wounds to be kept moist, the dressings to be well tolerated and the pain to be reduced while the integrity of the wounds was maintained during dressing changes. Fatty acids such as vitamin E represent a good option for debrided or cleaned wounds with good tolerance and ease of maintenance (GODOY; PRADO, 2005).

Manzi *et al.* (2003) evaluated the action of vitamin E as a
in the tissue repair process in rats. Analysis of the results showed that the delay in the tissue repair process caused by 6 Gy of electron radiation with a 6 MeV beam did not occur in the group of animals that received vitamin E, proving this substance to be effective as a radioprotector (MANZI *et al.,* 2003).

Studies have shown that oil from the fruit of *M. flexuosa*, a source of vitamin E, was effective in the healing process of cutaneous wounds in Wistar rats. It was able to promote a higher percentage of contraction of the wound edges and was statistically significant in the count of fibroblasts and collagen fibers in the group treated with buriti oil compared to the control group. *In* addition, they showed antibacterial activity *in vitro* against both gram-positive and gram-negative bacteria (BATISTA *et al.,* 2012).

In the study by Batista *et al.* (2012) Wistar rats were subjected to cutaneous wounds and treated with buriti oil. The results showed a significant reduction in the area of the wound on the 14th day and a higher percentage of wound contraction in the treated group compared to the control. On the 14th day, the wounds treated with buriti oil showed a significant increase in the count of fibroblasts and collagen fibres, as well as a complete re-epithelialization process, while the control group needed more time to resolve the healing process (BATISTA *et al.*, 2012).

3. CHAPTER 2 - OBJECTIVES

3.1 General

- Develop an explanatory booklet emphasizing the anti-inflammatory and healing effect of vitamin E.

3.2 Specifics

- Emphasize the anti-inflammatory effects of vitamin E.
- Emphasize the healing effects of vitamin E.
- Explain the mechanism of action of vitamin E on inflammation and the healing process.

4. CHAPTER 3 - METHODOLOGY

4.1 Type of study

This is a qualitative, bibliographic study based on scientific evidence of the participation of users of the health system. A creative approach was adopted, thus proposing the creation of an explanatory and illustrative booklet on the anti-inflammatory and healing effects of vitamin E.

The preparation of this educational booklet was based on information obtained through prior bibliographic research, where the researcher's initial step was to define the general objective guiding the booklet in order to answer and clarify the main doubts presented in the scientific literature on the subject.

According to Reberte *et al.* (2012) the use of dialogic strategies and
This is why the use of the booklet as an additional resource for very important educational activities, where the booklet's guiding objective is made clear right from the start.

4.2 Target audience

The educational booklet was produced with the aim of reaching a public of patients with diabetes, the elderly and bedridden individuals who are users of the PSF (Family Health Program). It is also useful as a scientific education and teaching-learning tool, which can be used by teachers, health professionals and academics.

4.3 Booklet construction process

4.3.1 Systematizing the content

The process of preparing an educational booklet on the importance of vitamin E was based on the principles of educational-dialogical practice. This process provides support for the possibility of helping users of public health services to change their lifestyle. Readers will have the opportunity to broaden their understanding of the problem and reflect on the intervention on the importance of using vitamin E (TORRES *etal.,* 2009).

The structure of the booklet was planned because of the need to use it in instructional interventions, communicating content with educational resources produced for health education. The growing use of educational materials enables the teaching-learning process. This brings challenges and requires clear definitions of the educational objectives to be presented to the target audience. The participatory approach used in the construction of educational material makes it possible to identify the needs of users, who indicate the content of the booklet corresponding to their own demands (OLIVEIRA *etal.,* 2014).

This work was based on the dialogic relationship and multidirectional principles, which allow for the existence of dialogue between those involved in the process of building a booklet. In turn, it was characterized by the identification of technical terms and their transformation into popular language, in order to make it easier for users to understand the booklet. Interaction and the exchange of knowledge, taking into account people's lifestyles, are essential aspects of successful work. Taking care to adapt the language to make it easier to understand is important in health education and promotion work. In this sense, we preferred to use popular words, especially colloquial ones (REBERTE *etal.,* 2012).

4.3.2 Selection and preparation of illustrations

The selection and use of some of the illustrations in the booklet is justified because, in many respects, they reproduce reality, reduce or enlarge the real size of the objects represented, bring facts and places distant in space and time closer together and allow for the immediate visualization of very slow or fast processes and facilitate understanding and comprehension by the target audience (RABELO *et al.,* 2015).

4.3.3 The composition of the booklet

At the stage of composing the booklet itself, contact was made with a professional in the field of communication, who was asked to edit the material. The content to be included in the educational material was passed on to this professional, who organized the images and we adapted the proposed script in a preliminary way that was indicative of a previous publication of the booklet.

5. CHAPTER 3 - RESULTS AND DISCUSSION

This booklet was developed taking into account bibliographical studies on vitamin E in texts and scientific articles, which are contained in the theoretical framework. The choice of topic was based on the importance of evaluating the use of an educational booklet to disseminate the use of vitamin E among patients with skin lesions. This study has demonstrated some of the beneficial effects of vitamin E in patients with various types of inflammatory processes. In addition, studies have shown the attraction and adherence of users to this type of educational material.

The booklet was designed using simple and relaxed language, in a didactic way, with the aim of avoiding too many pages, always aiming for the best understanding on the part of users, as well as the acquisition of knowledge about the subjects covered. In this way, it will become an important object, both for the health team, who will have simple material in their hands to complement their explanations when advising patients, and for the user, who will be able to take what they have been advised home with them and consult the information whenever necessary.

In terms of structure, the booklet is organized into (Cover, Back cover, Summary, Introduction, Getting to know vitamin E, Importance of vitamin E, Anti-inflammatory, antioxidant and healing effects of vitamin E, Sources of vitamin E, Vitamin E intake recommendations and Nutritious recipes). On the cover of the booklet is the theme "Super E", which with this approach I intend to draw the reader's attention to learn more about the information being offered in the booklet and to reproduce it in their daily lives.

The content of the booklet includes information about the importance of vitamin E, its effects and its support in the body. The language used was appropriate for the target audience, easy to understand and which, as well as informing, would bring pleasure and relaxation to the reader. The illustrative material included simple line drawings to make the content dynamic, interactive and attractive.

This study showed the importance of including foods rich in vitamin E, given its fundamental role in antioxidant, anti-inflammatory and healing processes.

In their study, Torres *et al.* (2009) reported that the development of educational booklets on topics relevant to users of the health system positively helps the process of health care and health professionals to take a relaxed and objective approach. In addition, it should create autonomy in individuals with regard to their health .

self-care and participating in conversations between professionals and their managers, with a view to resolving or addressing health problems.

Still in this context, Lima *et al.* (2014) makes us realize that health education becomes an important ally in the political pedagogical role, which contributes to users having a critical and reflective view, allowing these individuals to understand the environment in which they are inserted, transform their habits and increase their perception of the multiple factors that are linked to health.

In view of what has been discussed, it can be seen that health education is an educational process that emphasizes health knowledge, with the aim of bringing together users of issues that focus on the community, stimulating disease prevention, health promotion and the engagement of the population, and their participation, in matters related to health and quality of life (BRASIL, 2006).

In view of the above, the booklet seeks to attract its target audience to a perception in a peculiar way, driven by their need to knowledge about health and wound healing. The booklet is a way of facilitating access to health advice, helping users to learn more about vitamin E so that it can be included in their daily diet.

6. FINAL CONSIDERATIONS

The experience of producing the booklet showed that written material makes a valuable contribution to developing skills that favor individual autonomy. It is important to create, develop and produce quality materials that can meet the needs of users of the Family Health Strategy (ESF), always seeking to clarify doubts about the benefits and importance of using vitamin E on a daily basis.

This information booklet becomes an information tool in the health education process. It makes health learning a dynamic process, facilitating the work of health professionals and providing health service users with information on the care they need to ensure their health. It also highlights the importance of including foods rich in vitamin E in patients suffering from skin lesions and other chronic inflammatory processes. The booklet will support professionals, users and students in overcoming the doubts and difficulties that permeate vitamins and their antioxidant and anti-inflammatory functions, especially vitamin E, as well as its potential benefits.

The aim is that the educational experience using the booklet will be an important means of informing, building knowledge and promoting reflection on the benefits of vitamin E.

REFERENCES

ARAUJO, P. B. M.; BRANDAO, M. S.; CHAVES, M. H. Total Phenols and Antioxidant Activity of Five Medicinal Plants. **Quimica Nova**, v. 30, n. 2, p. 351-355, 2007.

AZZI, A.; GYSIN, R.; KEMPNA, P.; MUNTEANU, A.; NEGIS, Y.; VILLACORTA, L.; VISARIUS, T.; ZINGG, J. M. Vitamin E Mediates Cell Signaling and Regulation of Gene Expression, 2006.
DOI: 10.1196/annals.1331.009

BARBOSA, M. R.; SILVA, M. M. A.; WILLADINO, L.; ULISSES, C.; CAMARA, T. R. Plant generation and enzymatic detoxification of reactive oxygen species. **Ciencia Rural**, v. 44, n. 3, 2014.

BARREIROS, A. L. B. S.; DAVID, J. M.; DAVID, J. P. Oxidative Stress: Relationship Between Reactive Species Generation and Organism Defense. **Quimica Nova**, v. 29, n. 1, p. 113-123, 2005.

BATISTA, J. S.; OLINDA, R.G.; VITOR BRASIL MEDEIROS, V. B.; RODRIGUES, C. M. F.; OLIVEIRA, A. F.; PAIVA, E. S.; FREITAS, C. I. A.; MEDEIROS, A. C. Antibacterial and healing activities of buriti oil *Mauritia flexuosa* L.**Ciencia Rural**, Santa Maria, v.42, n.1, p.136-141,2012.

BERTAGNON, H. G.; SILVA, E. B.; CONNEGLIAN, M. M.; MIKAEL NEUMANN, M.; ESPER, G. V. Z.; BASTOS. G. P.; PEREIRA, J. R. Immunomodulatory action of vitamin E in systemic immunity and mammary gland of dairy cows fed silage. **Semina: Ciencias Agrarias, Londrina**, v. 35, n. 2, p. 857-866, 2014.

BERRA, A. S.; BARROS, C. R.; FERREIRA, S. R.G. Vitamins and minerals with antioxidant properties and cardiometabolic risk: controversies and perspectives. **Arquivos Brasileiros de Endocrinologia & Metabologia**, 2006. Available at:http://www.scielo.br/pdf/abem/v53n5/08.pdf

BIANCHI, M. L. P; ANTUNES, L. M. G. Free Radicals and the Main Dietary Antioxidants. **Revista de Nutrigao Campinas**, v. 12, n. 2, p. 123-130. 1999. Available at:http://www.scielo.br/pdf/rn/v12n2/v12n2a01.pdf

BRAZIL. Ministry of Health. Secretariat for Strategic and Participatory Management. Participatory Management Support Department. **Nutrition guide for patients and caregivers:** Guidance for patients. 2006.

BRAZIL. Ministry of Health. Secretariat for Strategic and Participatory Management. Participatory Management Support Department. **Caderno de educagao popular e saude. Brasilia: Ministry of Health**, 2007.

BRITO, M. V. H.; MOREIRA, R. J.; TAVARES, M. L. C.; CARBALLO, M. C. S.; CARNEIRO, T. X.; SANTOS, A. A. S. Copaiba oil effect on urea and creatinine serum levels in rats submitted to kidney ischemia and reperfusion syndrome. **Acta Cirurgica Brasileira**, v. 20, n. 3, 2005. *Available at: http://www. scielo. br/pdf/acb/v20n3/a09v20n3. pdf*

CABRERA, T. C; SERRANO, D. S. Algunos aspectos sobre el estres oxidativo, el estado antioxidante y la terapia de suplementacion. **Revista Cubana Cardiologia**, v. 14, n. 1, p. 55-60, 2000.

CERQUEIRA, F.M.; MEDEIROS, M.H.G.; AUGUSTO, O. Dietary antioxidants: controversies and perspectives. **Quimica Nova**, v. 30, N. 2, 441-449, 2007.

COSTA, N.M.B.; ROSA, C.O.B. **Functional foods - bioactive components**

and physiological effects - Part I - 3 antioxidant vitamins. Rio de Janeiro: Editora Rubio, 2010.

COZZOLINO, S.M.F. **Biodisponibilidade de nutrientes** - 3.ed.atual e ampl.- Barueri, SP: Manole, 2009.

COSTA, C. L. S.; ARAUJO, D. S.; CAVALCANTE, L. C. D.; BARROS, E. D. S.;

COSTA, T.; JORGE, N. Beneficial Bioactive Compounds Present in Nuts and Walnuts. UNOPAR **Cientifica Ciencias Biologicas e da Saude**, v. 13, n. 3, p. 195-203, 2011.

DIMENSTEIN, R; LIRA, L; MEDEIROS, A. C. P; CUNHA, L. R. F; STAMFORD, T. L. M. Effect of vitamin E supplementation on alpha-tocopherol concentration in human colostrum. **Revista Panamericana Salud Publica**, v. 29, n. 6, 2011. Available at: http://www.scielosp.org/pdf/rpsp/v29n6/03.pdf

FARFAN, J. A.; DOMENE, S. M. A.; PADOVANI, R. M. *DRI: Commented Note Of The New Nutritional RecommendaTions For Dietary Antioxidants.* **Revista de Nutripao Campinas,** v. 14, n. 1, 2001. Available at: http://www.scielo.br/pdf/rn/v14n1/7574.pdf

FILHO, G. B. BOGLIOLO**. General Pathology**. 4th Ed. Rio de Janeiro. Editora Guanabara Koogan S.A. 2009

FRANCO, G. **Tabela de composiQao quimica dos alimentos/** 9ª Ed. Sao Paulo: Editora Atheneu, 2008.

FERREIRA, R. J.; COTTA, R. M. M.; FRANCESCHINI, S. C. C.; RIBEIRO, R. C. L.; SAMPAIO, R. F.; PRIORE, S. E.; CECON, P. R. Contribution of the physical, social, psychological and environmental domains to the overall quality of life of the elderly, **Revista de Psiquiatria**, 2006.

FERREIRA, A.L.A.; MATSUBARA, L.S. Free radicals: concepts, related diseases, defense system and oxidative stress. **Revista Associapao Medicina Brasil,** v.43, n.1, 1997

GODOY, J. M. P.; PRADO, P. A. Essential fatty acids enriched with vitamin A, E and linoleic acid as dressings for chronic wounds. **Revista Portuguesa de Clinica Geral,** v. 21, n. 5, p. 193, 2005. Available at: *http://www. drenagemlinfatica. com.br/Ddfs/publicacoes/Acidos%20gordos%20essenciais.pdf*

GOLDMAN, L; AUSIELLO, D. **Cecil Medicina** [translated by Adriana PittellaSudre... *et al*]. - Rio de Janeiro; Ed. Elsevier, 2009.

GUYTON, A. C; HALL, J. E. **Test Book Of Medical Physiology**. 11th ed. Publisher ELSEVIER SAUNDERS. 2006

GUINAZI, M.; MILAGRES, R. C. R. M.; SANT'ANA, H. M. P.; CHAVES, J. B. P. Tocopherols and Tocotrienois in Vegetable Oils and Eggs. **Quimica Nova**, v. 32, n. 8, p. 2098-2103, 2009. Available at: http://www.scielo.br/pdf/qn/v32n8/v32n8a21.pdf

JUNIOR, F.; TELO, D. F.; SOUZA,H. P.; NICOLAU,J.C.; HALPERN, A; JUNIOR, C.V.S. Obesity and Coronary Artery Disease: The Role of Inflammation, 2001.

JUNIOR, B. R.; MORAIS, O. L.; SILVA, J. B.; SOUSA, R. B. A construpao da vigilancia e preventpao das doenças cronicas não transmissiveis no contato do sistema unico de saude. **Epidemiol revis saude**, [online] 2005.

LEITE, H. P.; SARNI, R. S. Free radicals, antioxidants and nutrition Radicales libres, antioxidantes y nutricion. **Quimica nova**. Sao Paulo. 2003.

LIMA, R. R.; COSTA, A. M. R.; SOUZA, R. D.; LEAL, W. G. Inflamapao em doenpas neurodegenerativas. **Revista Paraense de Medicina**, v. 21, n. 2, 2007.

LOPES, P. R. R.; CAMPOS, P. S. F.; NASCIMENTO, R. J. M. Pain and inflammation in temporomandibular disorders: a literature review of the last four years. **Revista de Ciencias Medicas e Biologicas**, v.10, n.3, p.317-325, 2011.

MANDELBAUM, S. H.; SANTIS, E. P. D.; MANDELBAUM, M. H. S.; MANHEZI, A. C.; BACHION, M. M.; PEREIRA, A. L. The use of essential fatty acids in the treatments of wounds La utilization de acidos grasos esenciales en el tratamiento de heridas. V. 78, n. 4, 2003.

MANZI, F. R.; BOSCOLO, F. N.; ALMEIDA, S. M.; TUJI, F. M. Mofologic Study of the Radioprotective Effect of Vitamin E (DL-alpha-tocopheryl) on Tissue Repair in Rats. **Radiologia Brasileira**, v. 36, n. 6, p. 367371. 2003.

MANHEZI, A. C.; BACHIONI, M. M.; ANGELA LIMA PEREIRA, A. L. The use of essential fatty acids in the treatments of wounds La utilizacion de acidos grasos esenciales en el tratamiento de heridas. **Revista Brasileira de Enfermagem**, v. 61, n. 5, p. 620-9, 2008.

MESSIAS, M. G. A Influência **de** Fatores Comportamentais e Ambientais Domesticos nas Quedas em Idosos; **Revista Brasileira de Geriatria e Gerontologia**, v. 12, n. 2, p. 275-282, 2009.

MONTERA, V. S. P. Benefits of Antioxidant Nutrients and their Cofactors for

Oxidative Stress and Inflammation Control in Heart Failure. 2007. Available at:http://www.vponline.com.br/downloads/artigo 1720.pdf

Monetta L. The importance of the nurse's scientific performance in the execution of dressings. **Revista Paulista de Enfermagem**, v. 9, n. 3, p, 83-7,1990.

MORAIS, D. C. M.; BARROS, P. O.; TAMOS, E. F.; ZUIM, N. R. B. Healing action of active substances: d-panthenol, sunflower oil, papain, propolis and fibroblast growth factor Foco, v. 4, n. 4, 2013.

MOURAO, M. O. F.; MOURA, J. B. F.; MANFREDINI, V.; BENFATO, M. S.; KUBOTA, L. T. Reactive Oxygen and Nitrogen Species, Antioxidants and Oxidative Damage Markers in Human Blood: Main Analytical Methods for their Determination. ***Quimica Nova,*** V. 30, 2005.

NOGUEIRA,C.; BORGES,F; ANDREA RAMALHO, *A.* Antioxidant micronutrients in neonates. **Revista Paulista de Pediatria**, v. 28, n. 4, 2010.

OLIVEIRA, S. C.; MARCOS, V. O. L.; FERNANDES, A. F. C.; SOUZA, S. C. O. Case study: Outpatient follow-up of patients with chronic renal failure. **Revista Latino-Americana de Enfermagem**, v. 22, n. 4, p. 611-20, 2014.

PAIXAO, J. A.; STAMFORD, T. L. M. Fat-soluble vitamins in foods - an analytical approach**. Revista Quimica nova**. 2004.

PENTEADO, M.V.C. Vitamins: nutritional, biochemical, clinical and analytical aspects. Sao Paulo: Manole, 2003.

PEREIRA, A. M. L.; VOGT, L. K.; CANAL, C. W.; LAGANA, C.; STRECK, A. F. Supplementation of Organic Vitamins and Minerals and their Action on the Immunocompetence of Broiler Chickens Subjected to Heat Stress. **Revista Brasileira de Zootecnia** , Vol. 37, 2009.

PHILIPPI, S.T. **Piramide dos alimentos**: fundamentos basicos da nutrigao - Barueri, SP: Manole, 2008. - (Nutrition and food guides). **Revista Brasileira Enfermagem**, v. 61, n. 5, p. 620 - 9, 2008.

PHILIPPI, S.T. Piramide dos alimentos: fundamentos da nutrição - Sao Paulo, SP: Manole, 2012. - (Nutrition and food guides). **Revista Brasileira de Enfermagem,** v. 61, n 5, p. 620 - 9, 2012.

RABELO, R. C.; GUTJAHR, A. L. N.; HARADA, A. Y. Methodology of the Elaboration Process of the Educational Booklet "The Role of Ants in Nature" Museu Paraense Emilio Goeldi. Belem - Para - Brazil. 2015

RAMALHO, V. C; JORGE, N. Antioxidants used in oils, fats and fatty foods. **Revista Quimica nova**. 2006

REBERTE, L. M.; HOGA, L. A. K.; GOMES, A. L. Z. The process of constructing educational material to promote the health of pregnant women. **Revista Latino-Americano de Enfermagem**, v. 20, n. 1,2012.

RIQUE, A. B.R.; SOARES, E.A; MEIRELLES, C.M. Nutripao e exercício na preventpao e controle das doenpas cardiovasculares. **Revista Brasileira de Medicina e Esporte,** v. 8, n. 6, 2002. Rio de Janeiro, RJ. Available at: http://www.scielo.br/pdf/rbme/v8n6/v8n6a06

ROITT, I. M.; BROSTOFF, A. J.; MALE, K. **Imunologia** 6° ed. Sao Paulo: Editora Guanabara koogan S.A, 2003.

ROITT, I. M.; DELVES, P. J. **Fundamentals of Immunology**. Ed. Sao Paulo: Editora Guanabara koogan S.A, 2004.

SALCI, M. A.; MACENO, P.; ROZZA, S. G.; SILVA, D. M. G. V.; BOEHS, A. E.; HEIDEMANN, I. T. S. B. Health education and its theoretical perspectives: some reflections**. Texto Contexto Enfermagem,** v. 22, n. 1, p. 224-30, 2013.

SAMPAIO, L. C.; ALMEIDA, C. F. Antioxidant Vitamins and Cervix Cancer Prevention. **Brazilian Journal of Cancerology**, 2009

SANTOS, H. S.; CRUZ, W. M. S. Oncologico the Antioxidant Vitamin Nutritionaltherapy and the Chemontherapy Treatment in Ongology. v. 53, n.1, p. 322, 2001. Available at:
http://ajcn.nutrition.org/content/53/1/322S.full.pdf+html

SCHNEIDER, C. D.; OLIVEIRA, A. R. Oxygen free radicals and exercise: mechanisms of formation and adaptation to physical training.

Revista Brasileira de Medicina e Esporte, vol.10, n.4, pp.308-313, [online]. 2004.

SILVA, W. D.; MOTA, I. **Imunologia Basica Aplicada**. 5th ed. Rio de Janeiro: Editora Guanabara koogan S.A, 2003.

SOUSA, C. M. M.; SILVA, H. R.; JUNIOR, G. M. V.; CRUZ, C. M.; AYRES, M. C. C.; SUCUPIRAA,N. R.; SILVA, A. B.; PEREIRA, G.; COSTA, J.N. Methods for Measuring Antioxidant Activity of Fruits 2007. UNOPAR **Cientifica Ciencias Biologica e da Saude**, v. 14, n. 4, p. 263-9, 2012.

SUCUPIRAA, N. R.; SILVAA, A. B.; PEREIRAA, G.; COSTAA, J. N.Methods for Measuring Antioxidant Activity of Fruits UNOPAR **Cientifica Ciencias**

Biologica e da Saude, v. 14, n. 4, p. 263 - 9, 2012.

TORRES, H. C.; FRANCO, L. J.; STRADIOTO, M. A.; HORTALE, V. A.; SCHALL, V. T. Avaliação Estrategica de Educapao em Grupo e Individual no Programa Educativo em Diabetes. **Revista de Saude Publica,** v.43, n.2, p.291-298. [online]. 2009.

VOLTARELLI, J. C.; Fever and Inflammation. In:. Medicina, Ribeirao Preto 1994. Anais Simposio: Semiologia e Fisiopatologia Clinicas. v. 27, n. 1/2, p 748, 1994.

VASCONCELOS, S. M. L.; GOULART, M. O. F.; MOURA, J. B. F.;MANFREDINI, V.; BENFATO, M. S.; KUBOTA, L. T. Reactive Oxygen and Nitrogen Species, Antioxidants and Oxidative Damage Markers in Human Blood: Main Analytical Methods for their Determination.
Quimica nova, v. 30, n. 5, p. 1323-1338, 2007.

ZINGG, J. M. This is the latest article added to the shopping cart. Vitamin E:An overview of major research directions.**Review Article Molecular Aspects of Medicine,** v. 28, n. 5-6, p. 400-422, 2007.

ZIMMERMANN, A. M.; KIRSTEN, V. R. Food With Antioxidant Function in Chronic Diseases: A Clinical Approach. **Quimica Nova**, v. 30, n. 5, p. 13231338, 2007.

APPENDIX 1

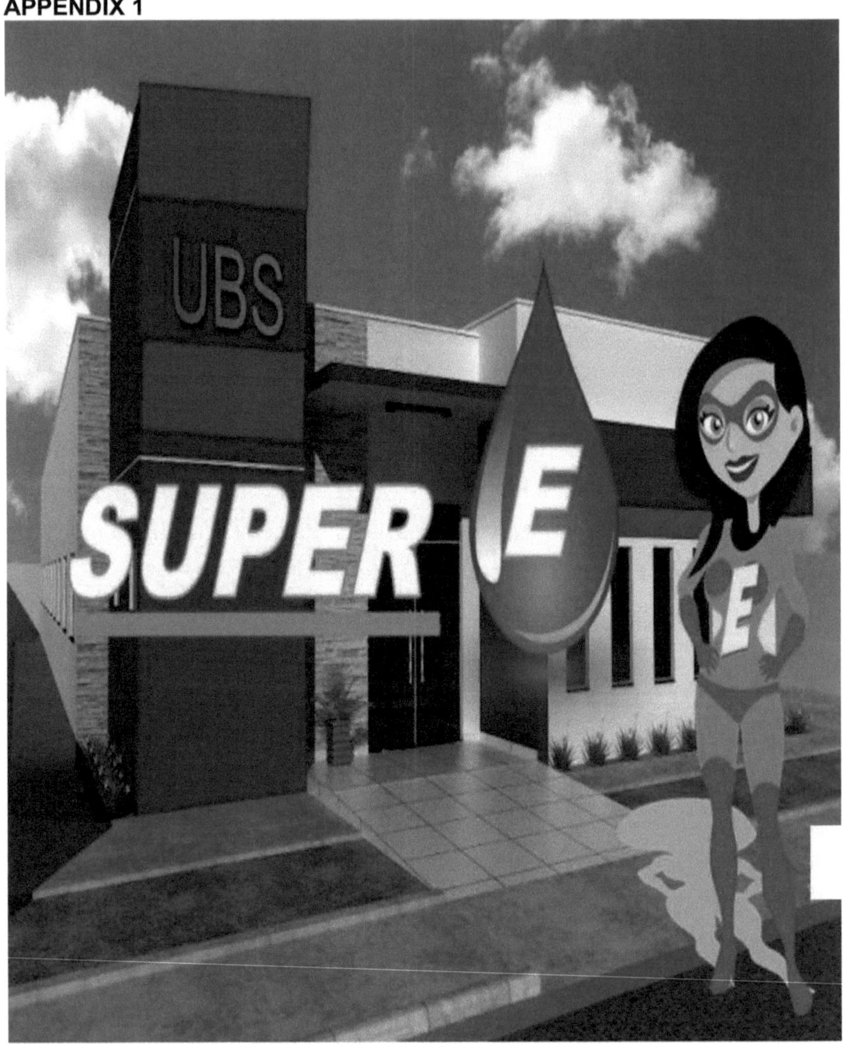

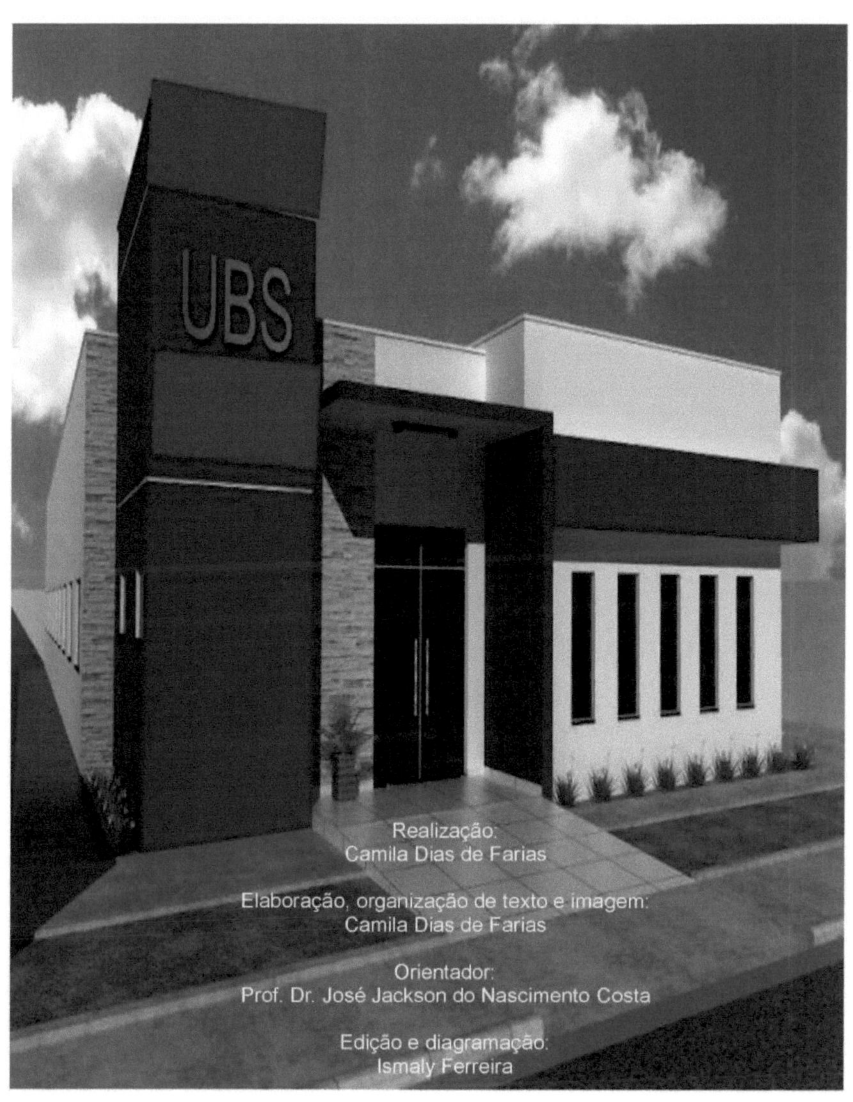
UBS
Realização:
Camila Dias de Farias
Elaboração, organização de texto e imagem:
Camila Dias de Farias
Orientador:
Prof. Dr. José Jackson do Nascimento Costa
Edição e diagramação:
Ismaly Ferreira

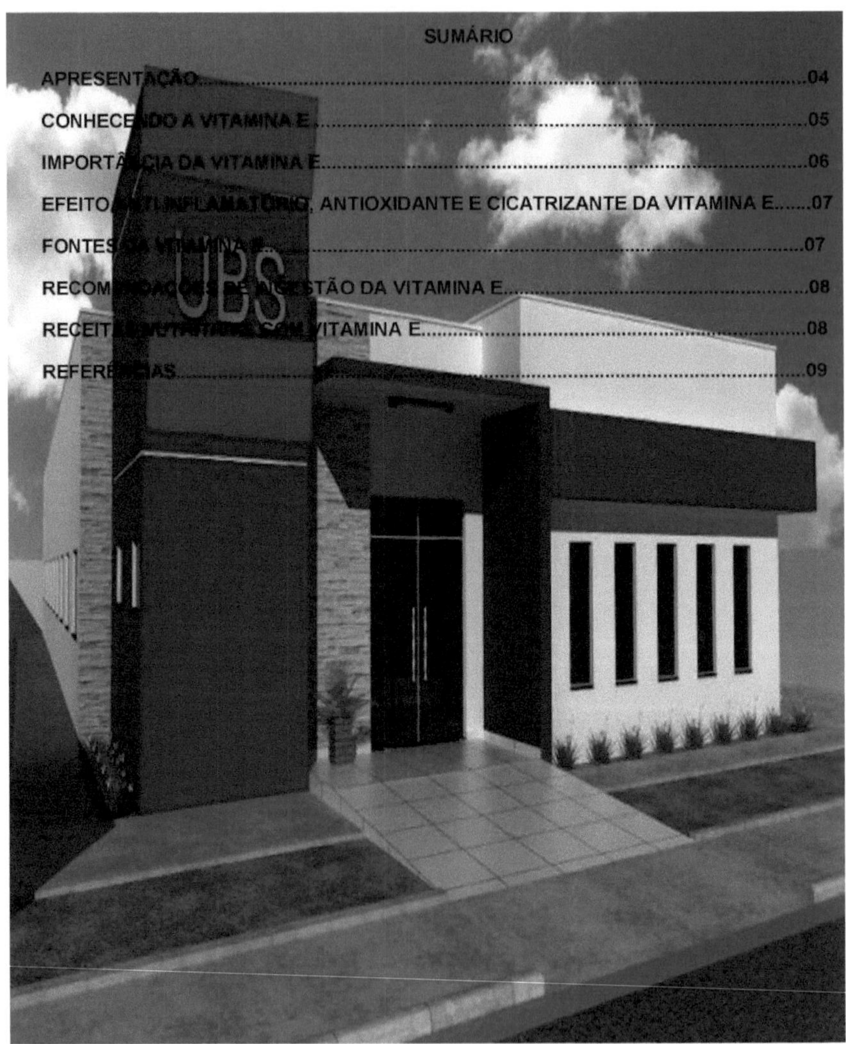

SUMÁRIO

APRESENTAÇÃO

Vitaminas são substancias orgânicas naturais, necessárias para o funcionamento normal das células vivas. A falta de vitaminas pode acarretar varias doenças.

A vitamina E ou tocoferol na natureza, identificam-se vários tipos de tocoferóis: alfa, beta, gama e delta. Popularmente é considerada a vitamina da fertilidade porque a sua função está diretamente ligada à produção de hormônios sexuais. Também é antioxidante, inibindo reações químicas que favorecem o envelhecimento celular e as doenças cardiovasculares. Desempenha funções antioxidantes sobre a vitamina A e os ácidos graxos insaturados. Dessa função, participa a vitamina C.

Protege os glóbulos vermelhos, evitando a anemia macrocítica comum em recém-nascidos desnutridos.

As melhores fontes da vitamina E são frutos oleaginosos como castanhas, nozes, amêndoas, azeite de oliva e óleos vegetais de soja, milho, entre outros. Alimentos de origem animal como carnes e ovos, são fontes secundárias. Em quantidades menores, aparece no germe dos cereais integrais.

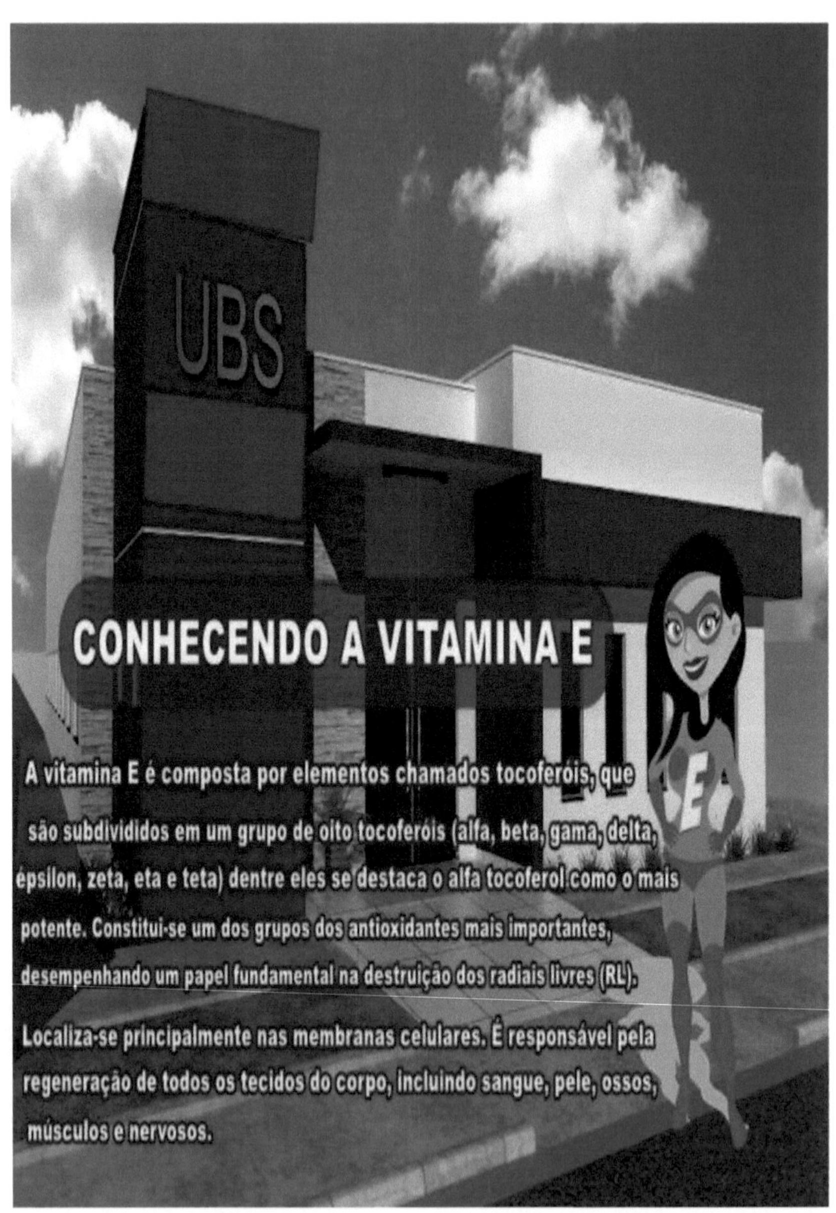
UBS
CONHECENDO A VITAMINA E
A vitamina E é composta por elementos chamados tocoferóis, que são subdivididos em um grupo de oito tocoferóis (alfa, beta, gama, delta, épsilon, zeta, eta e teta) dentre eles se destaca o alfa tocoferol como o mais potente. Constitui-se um dos grupos dos antioxidantes mais importantes, desempenhando um papel fundamental na destruição dos radiais livres (RL).
Localiza-se principalmente nas membranas celulares. É responsável pela regeneração de todos os tecidos do corpo, incluindo sangue, pele, ossos, músculos e nervosos.
E

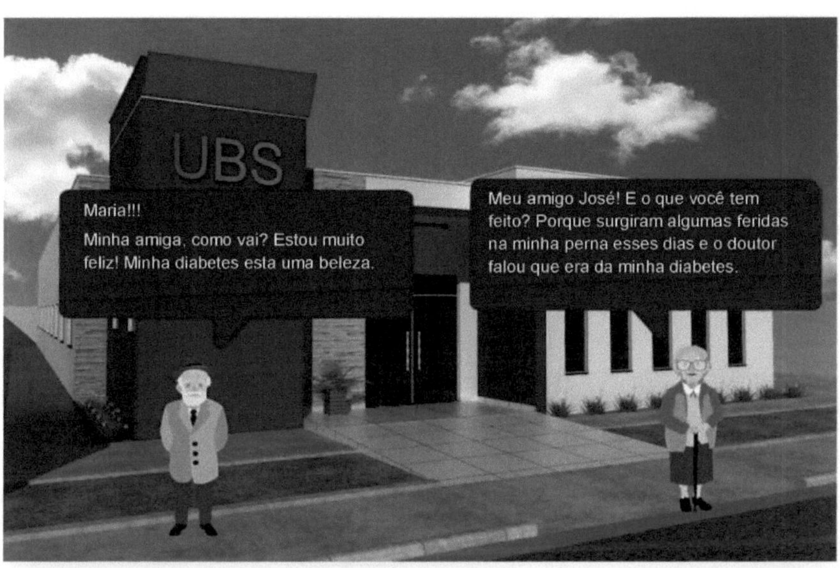
UBS
Maria!!!
Minha amiga, como vai? Estou muito feliz! Minha diabetes esta uma beleza.
Meu amigo José! E o que você tem feito? Porque surgiram algumas feridas na minha perna esses dias e o doutor falou que era da minha diabetes.

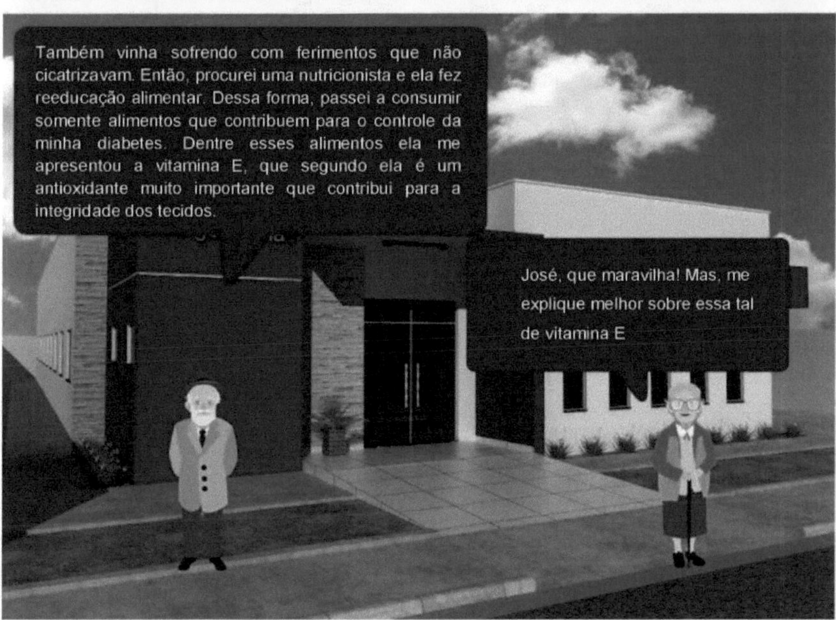
Também vinha sofrendo com ferimentos que não cicatrizavam. Então, procurei uma nutricionista e ela fez reeducação alimentar. Dessa forma, passei a consumir somente alimentos que contribuem para o controle da minha diabetes. Dentre esses alimentos ela me apresentou a vitamina E, que segundo ela é um antioxidante muito importante que contribui para a integridade dos tecidos.
José, que maravilha! Mas, me explique melhor sobre essa tal de vitamina E

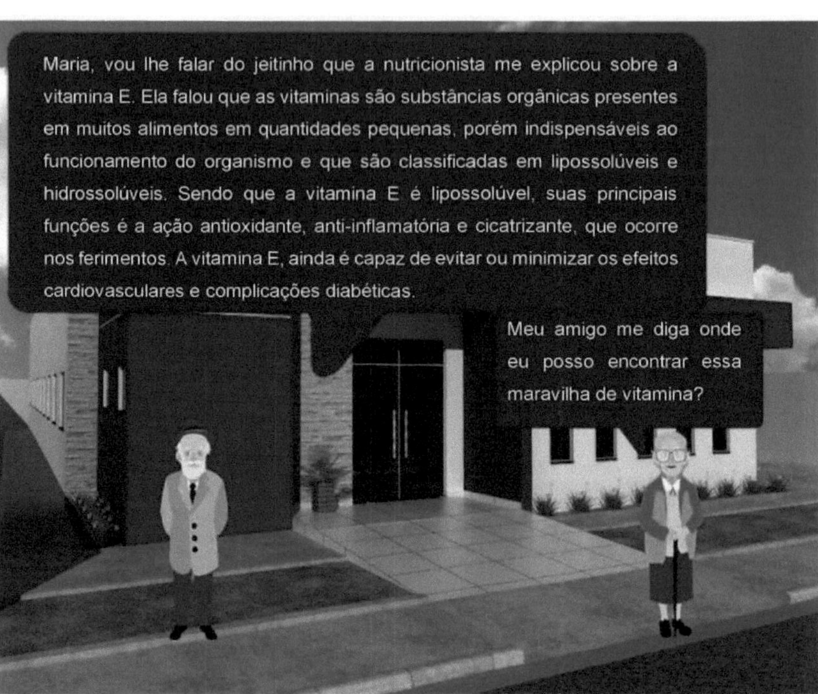
Maria, vou lhe falar do jeitinho que a nutricionista me explicou sobre a vitamina E. Ela falou que as vitaminas são substâncias orgânicas presentes em muitos alimentos em quantidades pequenas, porém indispensáveis ao funcionamento do organismo e que são classificadas em lipossolúveis e hidrossolúveis. Sendo que a vitamina E é lipossolúvel, suas principais funções é a ação antioxidante, anti-inflamatória e cicatrizante, que ocorre nos ferimentos. A vitamina E, ainda é capaz de evitar ou minimizar os efeitos cardiovasculares e complicações diabéticas.
Meu amigo me diga onde eu posso encontrar essa maravilha de vitamina?

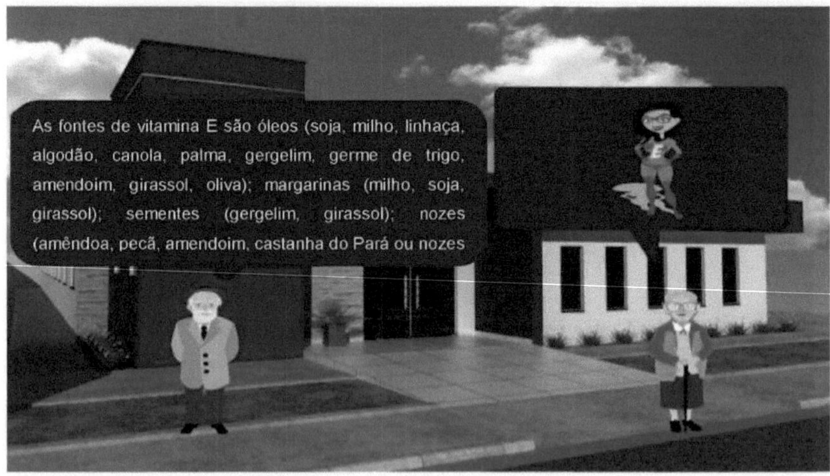
As fontes de vitamina E são óleos (soja, milho, linhaça, algodão, canola, palma, gergelim, germe de trigo, amendoim, girassol, oliva); margarinas (milho, soja, girassol); sementes (gergelim, girassol); nozes (amêndoa, pecã, amendoim, castanha do Pará ou nozes

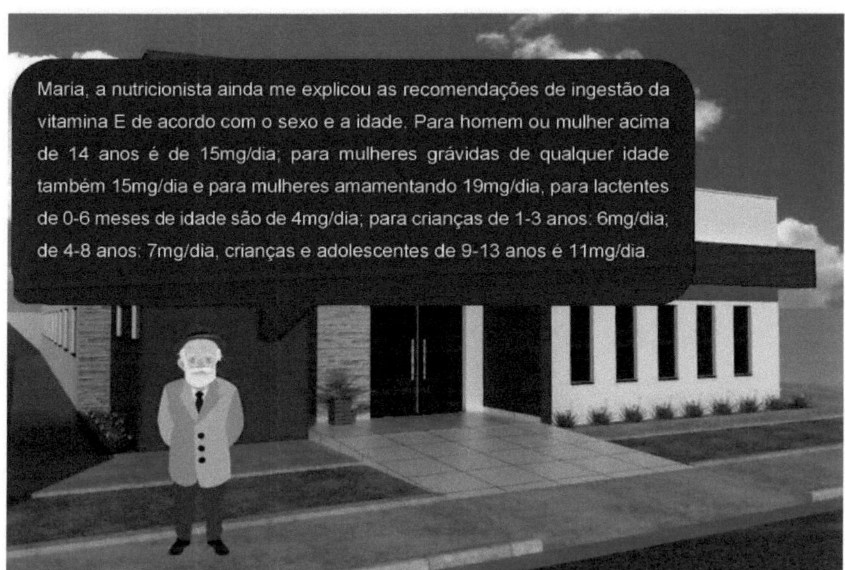

UBS
Veja aqui algumas receitas que são ricas em vitamina E.

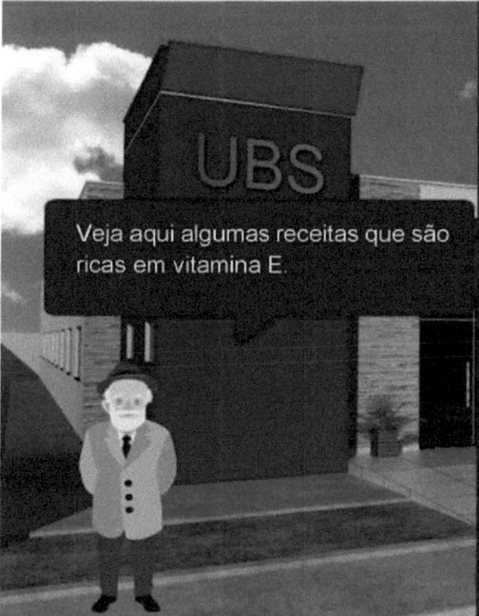

Purê de castanhas

Ingredientes

- 1 kg de castanha;
- 2 Col. de sopa da manteiga;
- 1 Xícara de leite quente;

Modo de fazer: Coloque as castanhas numa panela, cubra com água e deixe cozinhar por 30-40 minutos, ou até ficarem bem macias. Descasque as castanhas (se estiver usando castanhas ao natural) e reduza a purê batendo no liquidificador junto com a manteiga e o leite.

Mix de oleaginosas com frutas secas

30g a 40g de oleaginosas (nozes, castanhas do Pará e de caju, amêndoas, pistaches, amendoins, macadâmias, avelãs, nozes etc.)

2 ou 3 pedaços de frutas secas (uvas passas, damasco, tâmaras, figos secos, manga desidratada, abacaxi desidratado, maçã desidratada etc.)

BIBLIOGRAFIA

COSTA N.M.B; ROSA C.O.B. Alimentos funcionais – componentes bioativos e efeitos fisiológicos. Rio de Janeiro: Editora Rubio, 2010. Parte I – 3 vitaminas antioxidantes

COZZOLINO, S.M.F. Biodisponibilidade de nutrientes – 3.ed.atual e ampl.- Barueri, SP: Manole, 2009.

PENTEADO, M.V.C. Vitaminas: aspectos nutricionais, bioquímicos, clínicos e analíticos. São Paulo: Manole, 2003.

PHILIPPI, S.T. Pirâmide dos alimentos: fundamentos básicos da nutrição – Barueri, SP: Manole, 2008. – (Guias de nutrição e alimentação). Rev Bras Enferm, Brasília 2008 set-out; 61(5): 620-9. Disponível em: http://www.scielo.br/pdf/reben/v61n5/a15v61n5.pdf

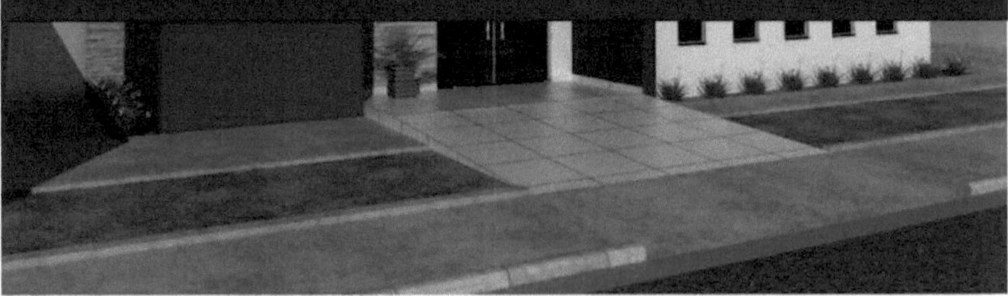

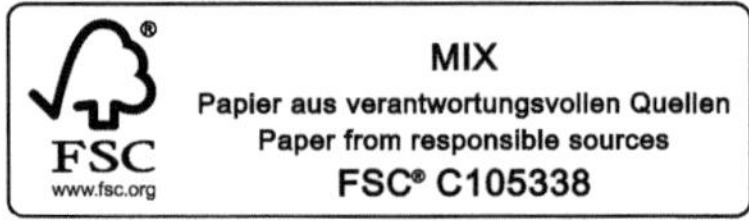

Printed by Books on Demand GmbH, Norderstedt / Germany